Mediterranean

Cookbook

365 Days of Healthy Recipes for a Balanced Diet! Colored Images and 14-Days Meal Plan Included

Sophia Scott

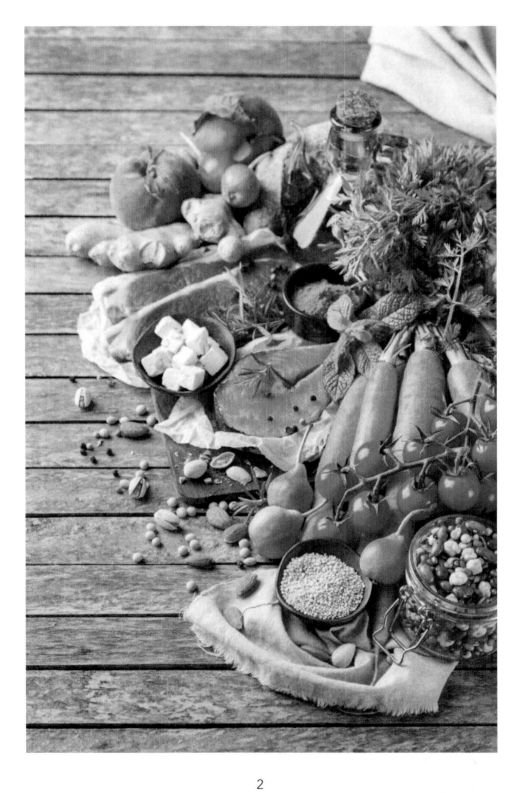

TABLE OF CONTENTS

INTRODUCTION

The Mediterranean diet is based on the foods eaten in countries bordering the Mediterranean Sea, such as Spain, France, Greece, and Italy

The word "diet" is often associated with an extreme or unpleasant way of eating. However, while it is called a "diet," it is not the classic stereotypical diet that you might follow to lose weight. Instead, it is a way of living and forms a vital part of the healthy Mediterranean lifestyle.

The Mediterranean diet varies from country to country, but each region follows the same basic principles.

WHAT ARE THE FUNDAMENTALS OF THE MEDITERRANEAN DIET?

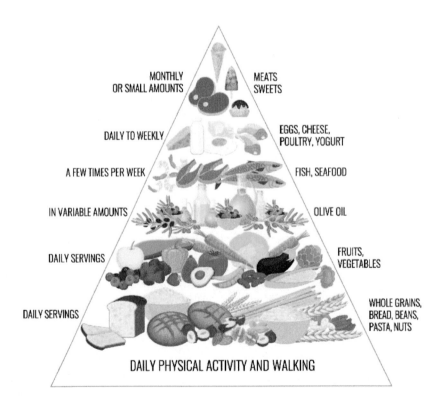

MONTHLY OR SMALL AMOUNTS — MEATS SWEETS

DAILY TO WEEKLY — EGGS, CHEESE, POULTRY, YOGURT

A FEW TIMES PER WEEK — FISH, SEAFOOD

IN VARIABLE AMOUNTS — OLIVE OIL

DAILY SERVINGS — FRUITS, VEGETABLES

DAILY SERVINGS — WHOLE GRAINS, BREAD, BEANS, PASTA, NUTS

DAILY PHYSICAL ACTIVITY AND WALKING

FOODS TO EAT

At the base of the pyramid are placed foods that make up a large part of the diet which include:
- Fruits
- Vegetables
- Whole grains
- Nuts
- Beans
- Legumes

The top portion of the pyramid represents the foods and drinks that are consumed in lower amounts, and this includes:
- Poultry
- Fish
- Healthy fats, such as those found in olive oil
- Some dairy products, such as eggs, cheese, and yoghurt

The pyramid's apex shows the foods eaten in tiny amounts, such as red meats and sweets.

Many diagrams of the Mediterranean diet also include a section for physical activity and social eating at the very base of the triangle.

FOODS TO AVOID

Things to avoid in the Mediterranean diet include highly processed foods that contain large amounts of saturated fat, sugar or salt.

MEDITERRANEAN DIET RULES

Eat high volumes of fruits, vegetables, beans, legumes, and whole grains. Since the base of the Mediterranean diet pyramid consists of all of these foods, it's important to consume each of them in every meal. Aim to include a range of different types of each category to maximize your nutrient intake and keep your diet fun and varied.

Consume lots of healthy fats, mainly by replacing butter with olive oil, and eat lots of nuts and seeds.

Eat moderate amounts of dairy and eggs, such as eggs, milk, and yogurt. Dairy is healthy in small doses, as it can help provide essential nutrients and strengthen bones. It can also lower the risk of cardiovascular disease, metabolic syndrome, obesity, and type 2 diabetes. However, excessive consumption of dairy products could cause health damage, so try to include dairy products in only two of your three daily meals.

Limit your intake of red meats and, instead, eat lots of lean meats, such as poultry and fish. Consumption of red meat has been linked to an increased risk of heart disease and poor digestive health. Red meat should be eaten in the Mediterranean diet no more than twice a week.

It is strongly suggested to eliminate highly processed foods. Try to reduce the amount of fast food and takeaway food you consume. Even better, eliminate them from your diet altogether. Instead, cook your own meals and snacks from scratch using healthy ingredients. It's also important to limit the amount of packaged or pre-made ready meals that you eat.

Drink lots of water and occasionally drink red wine. Water keeps you hydrated and aids digestion. Red wine contains resveratrol that reduces oxidative damage and inflammation in the body. You should also keep your consumption of high-calorie or high-sugar drinks to a minimum.

WHY THE MEDITERRANEAN IS SO FAMOUS?

The Mediterranean diet initially gained popularity back in the 1950s because researchers noticed that those who lived in Mediterranean countries, and, therefore, followed a Mediterranean diet seemed to have a lower incidence of heart disease.

Since then, further research has confirmed that the Mediterranean diet can promote good health, extend lifespan, and reduce the risk of heart attacks, strokes, type 2 diabetes, and premature death.

TUNA SALAD

10 minutes

0 minutes

2-4

INGREDIENTS

- 1 can (140 g) albacore tuna, solid white
- 1 to 2 tablespoons mayo or Greek yogurt
- 1 whole-wheat crackers
- 32 g chickpeas, rinsed, drained (or preferred white beans)
- 32 g Kalamata olives, quartered
- 32 g roughly chopped marinated artichoke hearts

DIRECTIONS

1. Flake the tuna out of the can into medium-sized bowl.
2. Add the chickpeas, olives, and artichoke hearts; toss to combine.
3. Add mayo or Greek yogurt according to your taste; stir until well combined.
4. Spoon the salad mixture onto crackers; serve.

Nutrition: Calories 105, Fat 2.5 g, Protein 11.5 g, Carbs 8 g, Fiber 1.5 g, Sugar 1 g

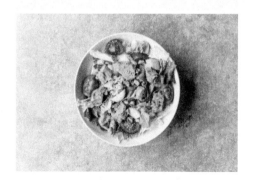

MEDITERRANEAN OMELET

3 minutes

10 minutes

1

INGREDIENTS

- 2 TB. extra-virgin olive oil
- 2 TB. yellow onion, finely chopped
- 1 clove garlic, small, minced
- 1/2 tsp. salt
- 128 g of fresh spinach, chopped
- 1/2 medium tomato, diced
- 2 eggs, large
- 2 TB. of whole or 2 percent milk
- 4 kalamata olives, pitted and chopped
- 1/2 tsp. of ground black pepper
- 3 TB. of crumbled feta cheese
- 1 TB. of fresh parsley, finely chopped

DIRECTIONS

1. In a nonstick pan, over medium heat, cook the extra-virgin olive oil, garlic, and yellow onion for 3 minutes.
2. Add salt, spinach, tomato, and cook for 4 minutes.
3. In a small bowl, whisk now together eggs whole milk.
4. Add the kalamata olives and black pepper to the pan, and pour in eggs over sautéed vegetables.
5. Using a rubber spatula, slowly push down the edges of the eggs, letting the raw egg form a new layer, continue for about 2 minutes or until eggs are cooked.
6. Fold the omelet in half, and now slide onto a plate. Now top with feta cheese and fresh parsley, serve warm.

Nutrition: Calories 466, Fat 36 g, Protein 17 g, Carbs 16 g, Fiber 6 g, Sugar 8 g

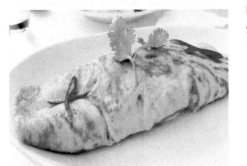

SALMON FRITTATA

 5 minutes

 27 minutes

 4

INGREDIENTS

- 450 g gold potatoes, roughly cubed
- 1 tablespoon olive oil
- 2 salmon fillets, skinless and boneless
- 8 eggs, whisked
- 1 teaspoon mint, chopped

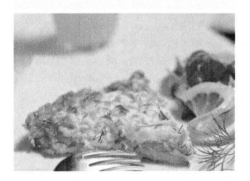

DIRECTIONS

1. Put the potatoes in boiling water at medium heat, then cook for 12 min, drain and transfer to a bowl.
2. Spread the salmon on a baking sheet lined with parchment paper, grease with cooking spray, broil at medium-high heat for 10 min on both sides, cool down, flake and put in a separate bowl.
3. Warm up a pan with the oil over medium heat, add the potatoes, salmon, and the rest of the ingredients excluding the eggs and toss.
4. Add the eggs on top, put the lid on and cook over medium heat for 10 min.
5. Divide the salmon between plates and serve.

Nutrition: Calories 330, Fat 16 g, Protein 24.5 g, Carbs 20 g, Fiber 2 g, Sugar 1 g

FETA AND ROASTED RED PEPPER BRUSCHETTA

5 minutes

15 minutes

24

INGREDIENTS

- 6 Kalamata olives, chopped
- 2 tablespoons green onion, minced
- 32 g Parmesan cheese, grated
- 32 ml extra-virgin olive oil
- 32 g cherry tomatoes, thinly sliced
- 1 teaspoon lemon juice
- 1 tablespoon extra-virgin olive oil
- 1 tablespoon basil pesto
- 1 red bell pepper, halved, seeded
- 1 piece (30 cm) whole-wheat baguette, cut into 1.5-cm thick slices
- 1 package (115 g) feta cheese with basil and sun-dried tomatoes, crumbled
- 1 clove garlic, minced

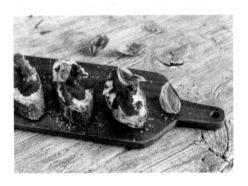

DIRECTIONS

1. Preheat the oven broiler. Place the oven rack 15 cm from the source of heat.
2. Brush both sides of the baguette slices, with the 32 ml of olive oil. Arrange the bread slices on a baking sheet; toast for about 1 minute each side, carefully watching to avoid burning. Remove the toasted slices, transferring into another baking sheet.
3. With the cut sides down, place the red peppers in a baking sheet; broil for about 8 to 10 minutes or until the skin is charred and blistered. Transfer the roasted peppers into a bowl; cover with plastic wrap. Let cool, remove the charred skin. Discard skin and chop the roasted peppers.
4. In a bowl, mix the roasted red peppers, cherry tomatoes, feta cheese, green onion, olives, pesto, 1 tablespoon olive oil, garlic, and lemon juice.
5. Top each bread with 1 tablespoon of the roasted pepper mix, sprinkle lightly with the Parmesan cheese.
6. Return the baking sheet with the topped bruschetta; broil for about 1-2 minutes or until the topping is lightly browned.

Nutrition: Calories 50, Fat 3.5 g, Protein 1.5 g, Carbs 3 g, Fiber 0.5 g, Sugar 0.5 g

ZUCCHINI CAKES

5 minutes

10 minutes

4

INGREDIENTS

- 1 zucchini, grated
- ¼ carrot, grated
- ¼ onion, minced
- 1 teaspoon minced garlic
- 3 tablespoons coconut flour
- 1 teaspoon Italian seasonings
- 1 egg, beaten
- 1 teaspoon coconut oil

DIRECTIONS

1. In the mixing bowl combine together grated zucchini, carrot, minced onion, and garlic.
2. Add coconut flour, Italian seasoning, and egg.
3. Stir the mass until homogenous.
4. Heat up coconut oil in the skillet.
5. Place the small zucchini fritters in the hot oil. Make them with the help of the spoon.
6. Roast the zucchini fritters for 4 minutes from each side.

Nutrition: Calories 65.6, Fat 1.5 g, Protein 3.5 g, Carbs 9.5 g, Fiber 1.5 g, Sugar 0.7 g

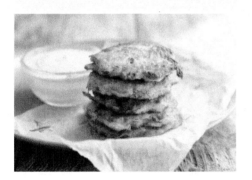

LEMON SALMON ROLLS

15 minutes   0 minutes   6

INGREDIENTS

- 6 wonton wrappers
- 200 g salmon, grilled
- 6 lettuce leaves
- 1 carrot, peeled
- 1 cucumber, trimmed
- 1 tablespoon lemon juice
- 1 teaspoon olive oil
- ¼ teaspoon dried oregano

DIRECTIONS

1. Cut the carrot and cucumber onto the wedges.
2. Then chop the grilled salmon.
3. Arrange the salmon, carrot and cucumber wedges, and lettuce leaves on 6 wonton wraps.
4. In the shallow bowl whisk together dried oregano, olive oil, and lemon juice.
5. Sprinkle the roll mixture with oil dressing and wrap.

Nutrition: Calories 133, Fat 2 g, Protein 8.5 g, Carbs 18.5 g, Fiber 0.5 g, Sugar 0 g

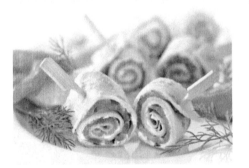

STUFFED AVOCADO

10 minutes

0 minutes

2

INGREDIENTS

- 1 avocado, halved and pitted
- 285 g canned tuna, drained
- 2 tablespoons of chopped sun-dried tomatoes
- 1 and ½ tablespoon basil pesto
- 2 tablespoons of black olives, pitted and chopped
- Salt and black pepper to the taste
- 2 teaspoons of pine nuts, toasted and chopped
- 1 tablespoon of basil, chopped

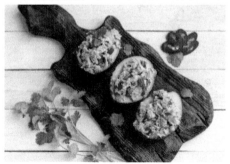

DIRECTIONS

1. In a bowl, combine the tuna with your sun-dried tomatoes and the rest of the ingredients except the avocado and stir.
2. Stuff your avocado halves with tuna mix.

Nutrition: Calories 350, Fat 17 g, Protein 36.5 g, Carbs 10 g, Fiber 5 g, Sugar 3.5 g

PARMESAN EGGPLANT BITES

 10 minutes

 30 minutes

 8

INGREDIENTS

- 2 eggs, beaten
- 85 g Parmesan, grated
- 1 tablespoon coconut flakes
- ½ teaspoon ground paprika
- 1 teaspoon salt
- 2 eggplants, trimmed

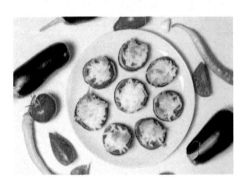

DIRECTIONS

1. Slice the eggplants into thin circles. Use the vegetable slicer for this step.
2. Sprinkle the vegetables with salt and mix them up. Leave them for 5-10 minutes.
3. Now drain eggplant juice and sprinkle them with ground paprika.
4. Combine together coconut flakes and Parmesan.
5. Now dip every eggplant circle in the egg and then coat in Parmesan mixture.
6. Line the baking tray with the parchment and place eggplants on it.
7. Bake the vegetables for 30 minutes at 180 C. Now flip the eggplants into another side after 12 minutes of cooking.

Nutrition: Calories 91, Fat 4 g, Protein 5.5 g, Carbs 8 g, Fiber 3 g, Sugar 4 g

PALEO ALMOND BANANA PANCAKES

5 minutes

10 minutes

3

INGREDIENTS

- 32 g almond flour
- ½ teaspoon ground cinnamon
- 3 eggs
- 1 banana, mashed
- 1 tablespoon almond butter
- 1 teaspoon vanilla extract
- 1 teaspoon olive oil
- Sliced banana to serve

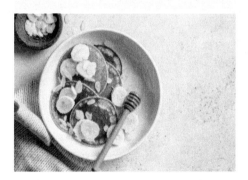

DIRECTIONS

1. Whisk eggs in a mixing bowl until they become fluffy.
2. In another bowl mash the banana using a fork and add to the egg mixture.
3. Add the vanilla, almond butter, cinnamon and almond flour.
4. Mix into a smooth batter.
5. Heat the olive oil in a skillet.
6. Add one spoonful of the batter and fry them from both sides.
7. Keep doing these steps until you are done with all the batter.
8. Add some sliced banana on top before serving.

Nutrition: Calories 182, Fat 7 g, Protein 8 g, Carbs 19.5 g, Fiber 2.5 g, Sugar 6 g

ITALIAN SCRAMBLED EGGS

5 minutes

7 minutes

1

INGREDIENTS

- 1 teaspoon balsamic vinegar
- 2 large eggs
- ¼ teaspoon rosemary, minced
- 64 g cherry tomatoes
- 192 g kale, chopped
- ½ teaspoon olive oil

DIRECTIONS

1. Melt the olive oil in a skillet over medium high heat.
2. Sauté the kale and add rosemary and salt to taste. Add three tablespoons of water to prevent the kale from burning at the bottom of the pan. Cook for three to four minutes.
3. Add the tomatoes and stir.
4. Push the vegetables on one side of the skillet and add the eggs. Season with salt and pepper to taste.
5. Scramble the eggs then fold in the tomatoes and kales.

Nutrition: Calories 174, Fat 9 g, Protein 14 g, Carbs 6 g, Fiber 0 g, Sugar 3 g

SPICED BREAKFAST CASSEROLE

10 minutes

30 minutes

6

INGREDIENTS

- 1 tablespoon nutritional yeast
- 32 ml water
- 6 large eggs
- 1 teaspoon coriander
- 1 teaspoon cumin
- 8 kale leaves, stems removed and torn into small pieces
- 2 sausages, cooked and chopped
- 1 large sweet potato, peeled and chopped

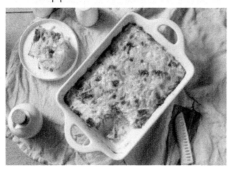

DIRECTIONS

1. Preheat the oven to 190 C.
2. Grease a 20 x 20 cm baking pan with olive oil and set aside.
3. Place sweet potatoes in a microwavable bowl and add 32 ml of water. Cook the chopped sweet potatoes in the microwave for three to five minutes. Drain the excess water then set aside.
4. Fry in a skillet heated over medium flame the sausage and cook until brown. Mix in the kale and cook until wilted.
5. Add the coriander, cumin and cooked sweet potatoes.
6. In another bowl, combine together the eggs, water and nutritional yeast. Add the vegetable and meat mixture into the bowl and mix completely.
7. Place now the mixture in the baking dish and make sure that the mixture is evenly distributed within the pan.
8. Bake now for 20 minutes or until the eggs are done.
9. Slice into squares.

Nutrition: Calories 137; Protein 10.1 g; Carbs 10.0 g; Fat 6.6g

CREAMY OATMEAL

3 minutes

15 minutes

2

INGREDIENTS

- 192 g oatmeal
- 1 tablespoon cocoa powder
- 64 g heavy cream
- 32 ml of water
- 1 teaspoon vanilla extract
- 1 tablespoon butter
- 2 tablespoons of Sweetener (Splenda)

DIRECTIONS

1. Mix up together oatmeal, cocoa powder, Splenda.
2. Transfer the mixture in the saucepan.
3. Add water, vanilla extract, heavy cream. Stir it now gently with the help of the spatula.
4. Close now the lid and cook it for 10-15 minutes over the medium-low heat.
5. Remove now the cooked cocoa oatmeal from the heat and add butter. Stir it well.

Nutrition: Calories 230; Fat 10.6; Fiber 3.5; Carbs 28.1; Protein 4.6

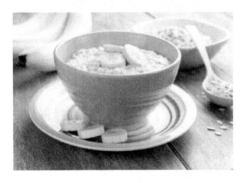

SUN-DRIED TOMATO PESTO PENNE

10 minutes

10 minutes

4

INGREDIENTS

- 226 g penne
- 64 g sun-dried tomatoes, drained well
- 2 tablespoons olive oil
- 4 garlic cloves, minced
- 2 tablespoons lemon juice
- 2 tablespoons pine nuts
- 2 tablespoons grated Parmesan cheese
- 1 pinch chili flakes

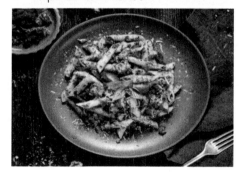

DIRECTIONS

1. Cook the penne in a large pot of salty water for 8 minutes or as long as it says on the package, just until al dente.
2. Drain the penne well.
3. For the pesto, combine the remaining ingredients in a blender and pulse until well mixed and smooth.
4. Mix the pesto with the penne and serve right away.

Nutrition: Calories 308, Fat:14.4 g, Protein:11.9 g, Carbohydrates: 34.1g

BROCCOLI PESTO SPAGHETTI

15 minutes

10 minutes

4

INGREDIENTS

- 226 g spaghetti
- 450 g broccoli, cut into florets
- 2 tablespoons olive oil
- 4 garlic cloves, chopped
- 4 basil leaves
- 2 tablespoons blanched almonds
- 1 lemon, juiced
- Salt and pepper to taste

DIRECTIONS

1. For the pesto, mix the broccoli, oil, garlic, basil, lemon juice and almonds in a blender and pulse until well mixed and smooth.
2. Cook the spaghetti in a large pot of salty water for 8 minutes or until al dente. Drain well.
3. Combine the warm spaghetti with the broccoli pesto and serve right away.

Nutrition: Calories 284, Fat 10.2 g, Protein 10.4 g, Carbohydrates 40.2 g

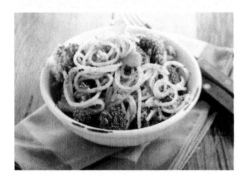

MEDITERRANEAN-STYLE TUNA WRAP

13 minutes

0 minutes

4

INGREDIENTS

- 1/2 teaspoon lemon zest
- 32 g fresh parsley, chopped
- 32 g Kalamata olives, chopped
- 32 g red onion, finely diced
- 2 cans (170 g each) chunk light tuna in water, drained well
- 2 large tomatoes, sliced
- 2 tablespoons lemon juice, freshly squeezed
- 3 tablespoons olive oil
- 4 whole-grain (about 55 g each) wrap breads
- 770 g mixed greens, pre-washed
- Freshly ground black pepper
- Salt

DIRECTIONS

1. In a medium mixing bowl, combine the tuna, parsley, onion, and olives.
2. In a small mixing bowl, whisk now the olive oil, lemon juice, lemon zest, salt, and pepper. Pour about 2/3 of the dressing over the tuna mixture; toss to incorporate.
3. In another bowl, combine the greens and the remaining 1/3 dressing; toss to coat.
4. Into each piece of wrap bread, top tuna salad, then with 64 g of greens, and a few slices of tomatoes. Roll the wrap; serve.

Nutrition: Calories 396, Fat 16.5 g, Protein 30 g, Carbs 31 g, Fiber 7 g, Sugar 7 g

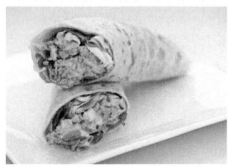

MEDITERRANEAN-STYLE SALMON BURGERS

15 minutes	4 minutes	4

INGREDIENTS

- 680 g skinless salmon fillet, cut into chunks
- 2 tsp Dijon mustard
- 2-3 tbsp minced green onions
- 120 g chopped fresh parsley
- 1 tsp ground coriander
- 1 tsp ground sumac
- ½ tsp sweet paprika
- 1/2 tsp black pepper
- Kosher Salt
- Breadcrumbs for coating, about 40 g or so
- 30 g extra virgin olive oil
- 1 lemon

Salmon Burger Toppings
- Tzatziki Sauce or Mayonnaise
- 170 g baby arugula more to your liking
- 1 red onion, sliced

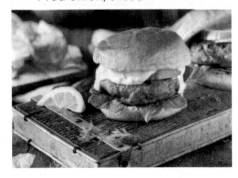

DIRECTIONS

1. Blend ¼ of the salmon together with the mustard until the mixture is pasty, then transfer to a bowl.
2. Blend the rest of the salmon so that it remains in pieces of about 0.5 cm; do not overblend it. Once you have completed the process, put it in the same bowl as before.
3. Add the chopped green onions, parsley, spices (cilantro, sumac, paprika, black pepper) and salt to taste . Stir everything together and then leave to chill in the refrigerator for about ½ hour.
4. While the salmon cools, prepare the toppings(wash the arugula, cut the tomatoes etc...).
5. Once the salmon has rested in the refrigerator, make 4 patties from the mixture.
6. Bread each patty in breadcrumbs and then arrange them on a baking sheet lined with baking paper.
7. Cook the patties in a frying pan with 3 tablespoons of oil for about 2-4 minutes. Be careful that the oil should already be hot before you start to cook the patties. The minimum internal temperature of the patties should be around 45-50 C to consider them cooked.
8. Once cooked, dry the excess oil well and season with additional salt and lemon juice if desired.
9. Now assemble the sandwiches by adding the tzatziki sauce (or mayonnaise) and garnish with the various toppings.

Nutrition: Calories 137, Fat 13.9 g, Protein 1 g, Carbs 4.2 g, Fiber 1.7 g, Sugar 0.9

TUNA PASTA

10 minutes

10 minutes

5

INGREDIENTS

- 350 g spaghetti (or pasta of your choice)
- Kosher salt (I use Diamond Crystal)
- 180 g frozen peas
- Extra virgin olive oil
- 1 red bell pepper, cut into strips
- 2 cans (140 g each) solid albicore tuna, drained
- Zest of 1 lemon
- Juice of ½ lemon
- Handful chopped fresh parsley (about 1 ounce)
- 6 garlic cloves, minced
- 1 tsp dried oregano
- Black pepper, to your liking
- 6 to 8 pitted kalmata olives sliced
- 1 jalapeno pepper, sliced
- Grated Parmesan cheese

DIRECTIONS

1. Boil 3 quarts of water and salt it. Cook the pasta according to the directions on the package so that it is al dente. After 5 minutes, add the frozen peas and cook them with the pasta for the rest of the time. Before draining the pasta, take some of the cooking water and set it aside(about 120 g).
2. Take a frying pan and heat two tablespoons of oil in it. Add the peppers and brown them for 3-4 minutes. The last 30 seconds, add the garlic.
3. Add the cooked pasta and peas to the pan and toss to combine. Pour in the rest of the ingredients and stir everything together. Add a little oil and use the cooking water to obtain a creamy consistency while stirring it.
4. Transfer the tuna pasta to serving bowls. Enjoy!

Nutrition: Calories 374.3, Fat 25.1 g, Protein 6.8g, Carbs 58 g, Fiber 5.1g, Sugar 3 g

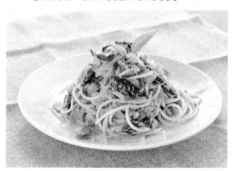

PARSNIP CHICKPEA VEAL STEW

10 minutes

2 Hours

10

INGREDIENTS

- 900 g veal meat, cubed
- 3 tablespoons olive oil
- 2 shallots, chopped
- 4 garlic cloves, chopped
- 2 red bell peppers, cored and sliced
- 2 yellow bell peppers, cored and sliced
- 4 parsnips, peeled and sliced
- 2 carrots, sliced
- 1 can diced tomatoes
- 192 ml beef stock
- 1 bay leaf
- 1 rosemary sprig
- 1 oregano sprig
- 1 can chickpeas, drained
- Salt and pepper to taste

DIRECTIONS

1. Heat oil in a heavy saucepan and stir in the veal. Cook for 5 minutes until slightly browned.
2. Add the shallots, garlic, bell peppers, parsnips and carrots.
3. Cook now for another 5 minutes then stir in the rest of the ingredients.
4. Season with salt and pepper and cook for 1 ½ hours on low heat.
5. Serve the stew warm and fresh.

Nutrition: Calories 332, Fat 12.7 g, Protein 27.8 g, Carbs 26.9 g

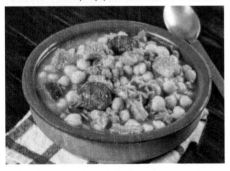

VEGETABLE RISOTTO

<30 minutes

10-30 minutes

4

INGREDIENTS

- 1 L stock broth (made with 1 vegetable or chicken stock cube)
- 1 large onion, chopped
- 2 medium carrots, cut into 1cm chunks
- 2 celery sticks, trimmed and cut into roughly 1cm chunks
- 3 tbsp olive oil
- 275 g rice for risotto
- 100 ml dry vermouth or white wine (optional)
- 2 pinches dried flaked chilies (crushed chilies)
- Lemon zest from 1 lemon, grated
- 2 garlic cloves, finely chopped
- 50 g grated Parmesan, plus extra to serve
- Salt and black pepper (optional)
- Chopped parsley, (optional)

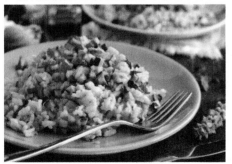

DIRECTIONS

1. Heat the oil in a large saucepan or medium flameproof casserole. Sauté the onion, carrots, and celery for 10 to 12 minutes, taking care to stir so they do not stick to the bottom of the pan. Toward the end add the garlic and cook for another 2 minutes.
2. Add the rice and toast it for 1 minute, stirring constantly (it should not stick). Deglaze with vermouth (or wine, if using) and evaporate the alcohol by cooking for 30-40 seconds.
3. Pour the stock and chili into the pot. Bring to a boil over medium heat and cook without a lid for 22-25 minutes, or until the rice is tender and very creamy. Stir the risotto every 4 to 5 minutes for the first 10 minutes of cooking, then more regularly as the liquid reduces and the rice swells; stir constantly for the last 5 minutes.
4. Once cooked, add the lemon zest and cheese. Season with salt and pepper and serve with more Parmesan cheese and chopped fresh parsley, if desired.

Nutrition: Calories 451, Fat 13 g, Protein 10 g, Carbs 64 g, Fiber 4 g, Sugar 7 g

CREAMY SALMON SOUP

5 minutes

15 minutes

6

INGREDIENTS

- 2 tablespoon olive oil
- 1 red onion, chopped
- Salt and white pepper to the taste
- 3 gold potatoes, peeled and cubed
- 2 carrots, chopped
- 500 ml fish stock
- 130 g salmon fillets, boneless and cubed
- 64 g heavy cream
- 1 tablespoon dill, chopped

DIRECTIONS

1. Heat a pan up with oil over medium heat, add the onion, and sauté for 5 minutes.
2. Add the rest of the ingredients expect the cream, salmon and the dill, bring to a simmer and cook for 5-6 minutes more.
3. Add the salmon, cream and the dill, simmer for 5 minutes more, divide into bowls and serve.

Nutrition: Calories 214, Fat 16.3g, Protein 11.8g, Carbs 6.4 g, Fiber 1.5g, Sugar 0 g

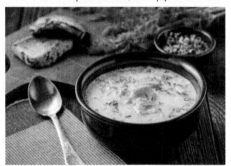

LAMB AND RICE

7 minutes

1 Hour and 10 minutes

4

INGREDIENTS

- 1 tablespoon lime juice
- 1 yellow onion, chopped
- 450 g lamb, cubed
- 30 ml avocado oil
- 2 garlic cloves, minced
- Salt and black pepper to the taste
- 256 g veggie stock
- 128 g brown rice
- A handful parsley, chopped

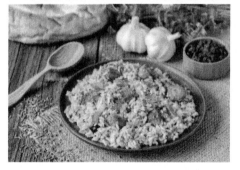

DIRECTIONS

1. Heat up a pan with the avocado oil over medium-high heat, add the onion, stir and sauté for 5 minutes.
2. Add the meat and brown for 5 minutes more.
3. Add now the rest of the ingredients except the parsley, bring to a simmer and cook over medium heat for 1 hour.
4. Add the parsley, toss, divide everything between plates and serve.

Nutrition: Calories 639, Fat 36 g, Protein 25 g, Carbs 50.5 g, Fiber 3 g, Sugar 3 g

ROSEMARY PORK CHOPS

5 minutes

35 minutes

4

INGREDIENTS

- 4 pork loin chops, boneless
- Salt and black pepper to the taste
- 4 garlic cloves, minced
- 1 tablespoon rosemary, chopped
- 1 tablespoon olive oil

DIRECTIONS

1. In a roasting pan, mix the pork chops with the rest of the ingredients, toss, and bake at 215 C for 10 minutes.
2. Reduce the heat to 175 C and cook the chops for 25 minutes more.
3. Divide the chops between plates and serve with a side salad.

Nutrition: Calories 539, Fat 35.5 g, Protein 51 g, Carbs 0 g, Fiber 0 g, Sugar 0 g

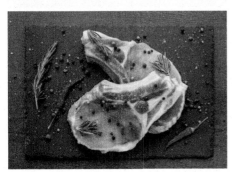

STUFFED PORK CHOPS

15 minutes

15-20 minutes

2

INGREDIENTS

- 1 beaten large egg
- Olive oil
- 1 very finely chopped shallot
- 40g spinach, blanched in boiling water and drained
- 30g chopped sun-dried tomatoes
- Finely grated zest of 1 lemon
- 1 crushed garlic clove
- 50g soft goat's cheese
- 2 bone-in pork chops
- 60g dried breadcrumbs
- Baby leaf salad and lemon wedges, to serve

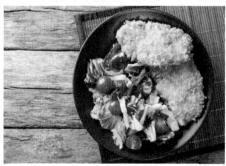

DIRECTIONS

1. Heat the oven to 180°C/160°C fan/gas 4. Heat some olive oil in a skillet over medium heat and sauté the chopped shallots for 5-6 minutes. Add the garlic and sauté for another minute then remove it. Add the blanched spinach, chopped sun-dried tomatoes, lemon zest and goat cheese with a pinch of salt and pepper and mix everything together.

2. Clean the pork chops by trimming the outer fat, then make a slit along the side of each chop to form a pocket. Stuff the pockets with the mixture prepared earlier. Bread the ribs by first dipping them in beaten egg and then in breadcrumbs.

3. Heat oil in a frying pan over medium heat and fry the pork chops for about 3 minutes on each side(they should be golden brown). Place the ribs on a small baking sheet and roast them in the oven for 15-20 minutes, until they are and cooked through.

Nutrition: Calories 610, Fat 36.4 g, Protein 46.5 g, Carbs 23.6 g, Fiber 0.9 g

HONEY PORK STRIPS

20 minutes

8 minutes

4

INGREDIENTS

- 285 g pork chops
- 1 teaspoon liquid honey
- 1 teaspoon tomato sauce
- 1 teaspoon sunflower oil
- ½ teaspoon sage
- ½ teaspoon mustard

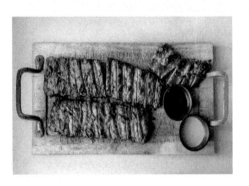

DIRECTIONS

1. Cut the pork chops on the strips and place in a bowl.
2. Add liquid honey, tomato sauce, sunflower oil, sage, and mustard.
3. Mix up the meat well and leave for 15-20 minutes to marinate.
4. Meanwhile, preheat the grill to 195 C.
5. Arrange the pork strips in the grill and roast them for 4 minutes from each side.
6. Sprinkle the meat with remaining honey liquid during to cooking to make the taste of meat juicier.

Nutrition: Calories 145.5, Fat 9 g, Protein 14.5 g, Carbs 0 g, Fiber 0 g, Sugar 0 g

BEEF PITAS

10 minutes

15 minutes

4

INGREDIENTS

- 192 g ground beef
- ½ red onion, diced
- 1 teaspoon minced garlic
- 32 g fresh spinach, chopped
- 1 teaspoon salt
- ½ teaspoon chili pepper
- 1 teaspoon dried oregano
- 1 teaspoon fresh mint, chopped
- 4 tablespoons Plain yogurt
- 1 cucumber, grated
- ½ teaspoon dill
- ½ teaspoon garlic powder
- 4 pita bread

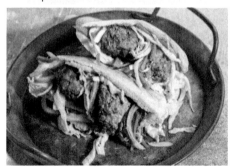

DIRECTIONS

1. In the mixing bowl combine together ground beef, onion, minced garlic, spinach, salt, chili pepper, and dried oregano.
2. Make medium size balls from the meat mixture.
3. Line the baking tray with baking paper and arrange the meatballs inside.
4. Bake the meatballs for 15 minutes at 190 C. Flip them on another side after 10 minutes of cooking.
5. Meanwhile, make tzaziki: combine together fresh mint, yogurt, grated cucumber, dill, and garlic powder. Whisk the mixture for 1 minute.
6. When the meatballs are cooked, place the over pitta bread and top with tzaziki.

Nutrition: Calories 264.5, Fat 6 g, Protein 14 g, Carbs 36 g, Fiber 1.5 g, Sugar 2.5g

LAMB AND AUBERGINE STEW

20 minutes

1.5 Hours

6

INGREDIENTS

- Olive oil for frying
- 750 g lamb neck fillet, cut into chunky strips
- 2 aubergines, halved and cut into strips
- 1 onion, finely chopped
- 5 dried figs, roughly chopped
- 3 garlic cloves, crushed
- 1½ tbsp baharat
- 1 tsp ground cumin
- 375ml hot chicken stock
- 125g mixed olives, roughly chopped
- Handful toasted flaked almonds
- Small handful each fresh mint, parsley and dill, coarsely chopped
- Pomegranate seeds
- Flatbreads to serve
- Hummus (page 68)

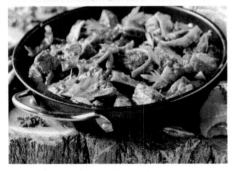

DIRECTIONS

1. Pour oil into a large, deep frying pan with a tight-fitting lid and heat it. Add the lamb, in batches, and fry it over high heat until golden brown. Once golden brown set it aside on a plate.
2. In the same skillet fry the eggplant; do not overcook it. Wipe off the oil in access once cooked and set aside on a plate.
3. Lower the heat and brown the onion (about 10 minutes). Add the figs, garlic, and spices and then cook for 2 minutes until fragrant.
4. Return the lamb to the pan and give it a stir then pour in the hot broth. Bring to a boil over high heat, then reduce the heat and simmer, covered, for 1 1/2 hours (the lamb should become tender). In the last 10 minutes of cooking, add the eggplant and 75 g of olives and stir so that the sauce thickens. Taste and season the stew with salt and black pepper.
5. Spread the houmous on the base of a large serving dish and pour the hot lamb stew over it. Decorate with the remaining olives, almonds, herbs, and pomegranate seeds.

Nutrition: Calories 568, Fat 32.9 g, Protein 37.8 g, Carbs 24.4 g, Fiber 11.4 g

PORK AND TOMATO MEATLOAF

10 minutes

45 minutes

4

INGREDIENTS

- 255 g ground pork
- 1 egg, beaten
- 32 g crushed tomatoes
- 1 teaspoon salt
- 1 teaspoon ground black pepper
- 30 g Swiss cheese, grated
- 1 teaspoon minced garlic
- 1/3 onion, diced
- 32 g black olives, chopped
- 1 jalapeno pepper, chopped
- 1 teaspoon dried basil
- Cooking spray

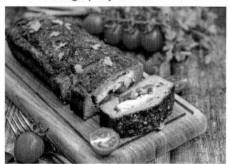

DIRECTIONS

1. Spray the loaf mold with cooking spray.
2. Then combine together ground pork, egg, crushed tomatoes, salt, ground black pepper, grated swiss cheese, minced garlic, onion, olives, jalapeno pepper, and dried basil.
3. Stir the mass until it is homogenous and transfer it in the prepared loaf mold.
4. Flatten the surface of meatloaf well and cover with foil.
5. Bake the meatloaf for 40 minutes at 190C.
6. Then discard the foil and bake the meal for 15 minutes more.
7. Chill the cooked meatloaf to the room temperature and then remove it from the loaf mold.
8. Slice it on the servings.

Nutrition: Calories 181, Fat 14 g, Protein 12 g, Carbs 0.5 g, Fiber 0 g, Sugar 0.5 g

CHICKEN QUESADILLA

12 minutes

20 minutes

4

INGREDIENTS

- 2 bread tortillas
- 1 teaspoon butter
- 2 teaspoons olive oil
- 1 teaspoon Taco seasoning
- 170 g chicken breast, skinless, boneless, sliced
- 42.5 g Cheddar cheese, shredded
- 1 bell pepper, cut on the wedges

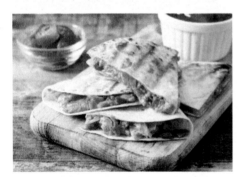

DIRECTIONS

1. Pour 1 teaspoon of olive oil in the skillet and add chicken.
2. Sprinkle the meat with Taco seasoning and mix up well.
3. Roast chicken for 10 minutes over the medium heat. Stir it from time to time.
4. Then transfer the cooked chicken in the plate.
5. Add remaining olive oil in the skillet.
6. Then add bell pepper and roast it for 5 minutes. Stir it all the time.
7. Mix up together bell pepper with chicken.
8. Toss butter in the skillet and melt it.
9. Put 1 tortilla in the skillet.
10. Put Cheddar cheese on the tortilla and flatten it.
11. Then add chicken-pepper mixture and cover it with the second tortilla.
12. Roast the quesadilla for 2 minutes from each side.
13. Cut the cooked meal on the halves and transfer in the serving plates.

Nutrition: Calories 176.5, Fat 10.5 g, Protein 13 g, Carbs 6 g, Fiber 0.5 g, Sugar 0 g

COCONUT CHICKEN

10 minutes

5 minutes

4

INGREDIENTS

- 170 g chicken fillet
- 32 g of sparkling water
- 1 egg
- 3 tablespoons coconut flakes
- 1 tablespoon coconut oil
- 1 teaspoon Greek Seasoning

DIRECTIONS

1. Cut the chicken fillet on small pieces (nuggets).
2. Then crack the egg in the bowl and whisk it.
3. Mix up together egg and sparkling water.
4. Add Greek seasoning and stir gently.
5. Dip the chicken nuggets in the egg mixture and then coat in the coconut flakes.
6. Melt the coconut oil in the skillet and heat it up until it is shimmering.
7. Then add prepared chicken nuggets.
8. Roast them for 1 minute from each or until they are light brown.
9. Dry the cooked chicken nuggets with the help of the paper towel and transfer in the serving plates.

Nutrition: Calories 139, Fat 9 g, Protein 12 g, Carbs 1.5 g, Fiber 1 g, Sugar 0.5 g

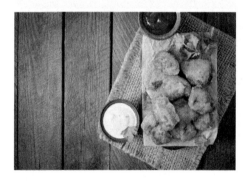

PARMESAN CHICKEN

10 minutes

30 minutes

3

INGREDIENTS

- 450 g chicken breast, skinless, boneless
- 60 g Parmesan, grated
- 1 teaspoon dried oregano
- ½ teaspoon dried cilantro
- 1 tablespoon Panko bread crumbs
- 1 egg, beaten
- 1 teaspoon turmeric

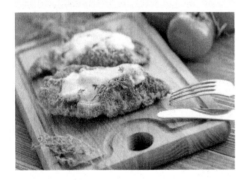

DIRECTIONS

1. Cut the chicken breast on 3 servings.
2. Then combine together Parmesan, oregano, cilantro, bread crumbs, and turmeric.
3. Dip the chicken servings in the beaten egg carefully.
4. Then coat every chicken piece in the cheese-bread crumbs mixture.
5. Line the baking tray with the baking paper.
6. Arrange the chicken pieces in the tray.
7. Bake the chicken for 30 minutes at 185 C.

Nutrition: Calories 378, Fat 19 g, Protein 38 g, Carbs 6.5 g, Fiber 0 g, Sugar 0.5 g

CHIPOTLE TURKEY AND TOMATOES

5 minutes

1 Hour

4

INGREDIENTS

- 900 g cherry tomatoes, halved
- 3 tablespoons olive oil
- 1 red onion, roughly chopped
- 1 big turkey breast, skinless, boneless and sliced
- 3 garlic cloves, chopped
- 3 red chili peppers, chopped
- 4 tablespoons chipotle paste
- Zest of ½ lemon, grated
- Juice of 1 lemon
- Salt and black pepper to the taste
- A handful coriander, chopped

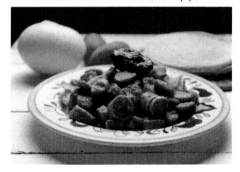

DIRECTIONS

1. Heat up a pan with the oil over medium-high heat, add the turkey slices, cook for 4 minutes on each side and transfer to a roasting pan.
2. Heat up the pan again over medium-high heat, add the onion, garlic and chili peppers and sauté for 2 minutes.
3. Add chipotle paste, sauté for 3 minutes more and pour over the turkey slices.
4. Toss the turkey slices with the chipotle mix, also add the rest of the ingredients except the coriander, introduce in the oven and bake at 200 C for 45 minutes.
5. Divide everything between plates, sprinkle the coriander on top and serve.

Nutrition: Calories 212.5, Fat 12 g, Protein 10.5 g, Carbs 14.5 g, Fiber 3 g, Sugar 11 g

BASIL TURKEY AND ZUCCHINIS

10 minutes

1 Hour

4

INGREDIENTS

- 2 tablespoons avocado oil
- 450 g turkey breast, skinless, boneless and sliced
- Salt and black pepper to the taste
- 3 garlic cloves, minced
- 2 zucchinis, sliced
- 128 g chicken stock
- 32 g heavy cream
- 2 tablespoons basil, chopped

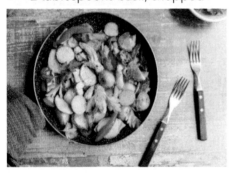

DIRECTIONS

1. Heat up a pot with the oil over medium-high heat, add the turkey and brown for 5 minutes on each side.
2. Add the garlic and cook everything for 1 minute.
3. Add the rest of the ingredients except the basil, toss gently, bring to a simmer and cook over medium-low heat for 50 minutes.
4. Add the basil, toss, divide the mix between plates and serve.

Nutrition: Calories 215, Fat 16 g, Protein 14 g, Carbs 14.5 g, Fiber 0.5 g, Sugar 1 g

BASIL CHICKEN WITH OLIVES

 10 minutes

 40 minutes

 5

INGREDIENTS

- 680 g chicken breast, skinless, boneless
- 3 Kalamata olives, chopped
- 1 teaspoon minced garlic
- 1 teaspoon salt
- 1 teaspoon ground black pepper
- 2 tablespoons sunflower oil
- 1 tablespoon fresh basil, chopped
- ½ teaspoon chili flakes
- 1 tablespoon lemon juice
- ½ teaspoon honey
- 32 ml of water

DIRECTIONS

1. Combine together Kalamata olives, minced garlic, salt, ground black pepper, sunflower oil, basil, chili flakes, lemon juice, and honey.
2. Whisk the mixture until homogenous.
3. Chop the chicken breast roughly and arrange it in the baking dish.
4. Pour olives mixture over the chicken.
5. Then mix up it with the help of the fingertips.
6. Add water and cover the baking dish with foil.
7. Pierce the foil with the help of the fork or knife to give the "air" for meat during cooking.
8. Bake the chicken for 40 minutes at 180 C.

Nutrition: Calories 288, Fat 18 g, Protein 29 g, Carbs 0 g, Fiber 0 g, Sugar 0 g

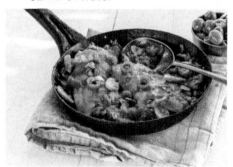

CHICKEN AND GRAPES SALAD

 15 minutes

 0 minutes

 4

INGREDIENTS

- 200 g chicken breast, skinless, boneless, cooked
- 64 g red grapes
- 30 g celery stalk, chopped
- 1 red onion, sliced
- 64 g Greek yogurt
- ½ teaspoon honey
- 1 tablespoon fresh parsley, chopped
- 1 cucumber, chopped

DIRECTIONS

1. Chop the chicken breast and place it in the salad bowl.
2. Add red grapes, celery stalk, sliced red onion, parsley, and cucumber.
3. Mix up the salad mixture.
4. Then mix up together Greek yogurt and honey.
5. Pour Greek yogurt mixture over the salad and stir well.

Nutrition: Calories 121, Fat 4.5 g, Protein 12 g, Carbs 7 g, Fiber 0 g, Sugar 5 g

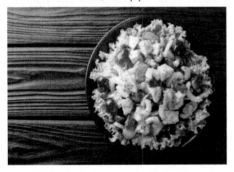

CORIANDER CHICKEN DRUMSTICKS

5 minutes

30 minutes

4

INGREDIENTS

- 8 chicken drumsticks
- 1 lemon
- 1 teaspoon minced garlic
- 1 teaspoon ground coriander
- 42.5 g onion, chopped
- ½ teaspoon ground turmeric
- 1 teaspoon paprika
- 1 teaspoon salt
- 1 tablespoon olive oil
- 1 teaspoon butter
- 42.5 ml water

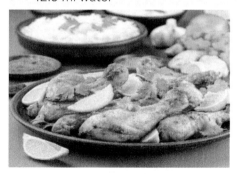

DIRECTIONS

1. Peel the lemon and chop the lemon pulp. Place it in the saucepan.
2. Add minced garlic, ground coriander, onion, turmeric, paprika, salt, olive oil, and butter.
3. Then add water and bring the mixture to boil. Mix it up.
4. Add chicken drumsticks and close the lid.
5. Simmer the chicken for 30 minutes over the medium-low heat.

Nutrition: Calories 420.5, Fat 41 g, Protein 11 g, Carbs 7.5 g, Fiber 0 g, Sugar 0.5 g

TURKEY, LEEKS AND CARROTS

15 minutes

45 minutes

4

INGREDIENTS

- 1 big turkey breast, skinless, boneless and cubed
- 2 tablespoons avocado oil
- Salt and black pepper to the taste
- 1 tablespoon sweet paprika
- 64 ml chicken stock
- 1 leek, sliced
- 1 carrot, sliced
- 1 yellow onion, chopped
- 1 tablespoon lemon juice
- 1 teaspoon cumin, ground
- 1 tablespoon basil, chopped

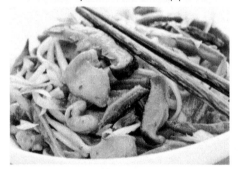

DIRECTIONS

1. Heat up a pan with the oil over medium-high heat, now add the turkey and brown for 4 minutes on each side.
2. Add the leeks, carrot and the onion and sauté everything for 5 minutes more.
3. Now add the rest of the ingredients, bring to a simmer and cook over medium heat for 40 minutes.
4. Divide the mix between plates and serve.

Nutrition: Calories 146.5, Fat 7 g, Protein 11.5 g, Carbs 7.5 g, Fiber 1 g, Sugar 3.5 g

SALMON AND MANGO MIX

5 minutes

25 minutes

2

INGREDIENTS

- 2 salmon fillets, skinless and boneless
- Salt and pepper to the taste
- 2 tablespoons olive oil
- 2 garlic cloves, minced
- 2 mangos, peeled and cubed
- 1 red chili, chopped
- 1 small piece ginger, grated
- Juice of 1 lime
- 1 tablespoon cilantro, chopped

DIRECTIONS

1. In a roasting pan, combine the salmon with the oil, garlic and the rest of the ingredients except the cilantro, toss, introduce in the oven at 175 C and bake for 25 minutes.
2. Divide everything between plates and serve with the cilantro sprinkled on top.

Nutrition: Calories 403, Fat 13.5 g, Protein 22 g, Carbs 50 g, Fiber 5 g, Sugar 45 g

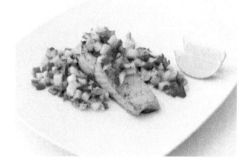

FRIED SALMON

5 minutes

8 minutes

2

INGREDIENTS

- 140 g salmon fillet
- ¼ teaspoon salt
- ½ teaspoon ground black pepper
- 1 tablespoon sunflower oil
- ¼ teaspoon lime juice

DIRECTIONS

1. Cut the salmon fillet on 2 lengthwise pieces.
2. Sprinkle every fish piece with salt, ground black pepper, and lime juice.
3. Pour sunflower oil in the skillet and preheat it until shimmering.
4. Then place fish fillets in the hot oil and cook them for 3 minutes from each side.

Nutrition: Calories 166, Fat 11 g, Protein 15 g, Carbs 0 g, Fiber 0 g, Sugar 0 g

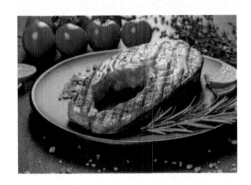

CORIANDER SHRIMPS

15 minutes

5 minutes

6

INGREDIENTS

- 1 hot chili pepper
- 32 g fresh coriander leaves
- ½ teaspoon ground cumin
- 2 garlic cloves, peeled
- ½ teaspoon salt
- 1 tablespoon lemon juice
- 2 tablespoons olive oil
- 900 g shrimps, peeled

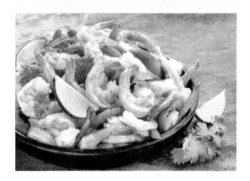

DIRECTIONS

1. Place in the blender: hot chili pepper, fresh coriander leaves, ground cumin, garlic cloves, salt, lemon juice, and olive oil. Blend the spices until you get the smooth texture of the mixture.
2. After this, place peeled shrimps in the big bowl.
3. Pour the blended spice mass over the shrimps. Mix up well.
4. Then preheat skillet well.
5. Place the shrimps and all spicy mixture in the skillet.
6. Roast the seafood for 5 minutes over the medium heat. Stir the shrimps with the help of the wooden spatula from time to time.
7. Then remove the shrimps from the heat and let them rest for 10 minutes before serving.

Nutrition: Calories 132.5, Fat 1 g, Protein 30 g, Carbs 1 g, Fiber 0 g, Sugar 0 g

SEAFOOD PAELLA

9 minutes

41 minutes

4

INGREDIENTS

- 4 small lobster tails (340 g each)
- 3 tbsp. Extra Virgin Olive Oil
- 1 large yellow onion
- 256 g Spanish rice
- 4 garlic cloves
- 2 large pinches of Spanish saffron threads
- 1 tsp. Sweet Spanish paprika
- 1 tsp. cayenne pepper
- 1/2 tsp. Aleppo pepper flakes
- 2 large Roma tomatoes
- 170 g. French green beans
- 450 g prawns or large shrimp
- 32 g chopped fresh parsley

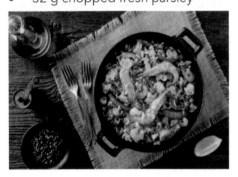

DIRECTIONS

1. Using big pot, add 385 ml of water and bring it to a rolling boil
2. Add in the lobster tails and allow boil briefly, about 1-min or until pink, remove from heat
3. Using tongs situate the lobster tails to a plate and do not discard the lobster cooking water
4. Allow the lobster to cool, then remove the shell and cut into large chunks.
5. Using a deep pan or skillet over medium-high heat, add 3 tbsp olive oil
6. Add the chopped onions, sauté the onions for 2 min and then add the rice, and cook for 3 more min, stirring regularly
7. Then add in the lobster cooking water and the chopped garlic and, stir in the saffron and its soaking liquid, cayenne pepper, Aleppo pepper, paprika, and salt
8. Gently stir in the chopped tomatoes and green beans, bring to a boil and allow it to slightly reduce, then cover and cook over low heat for 20 min
9. Once done, uncover and spread the shrimp over the rice, push it into the rice slightly, add in a little water, if needed
10. Close and cook for 18 min
11. Then add in the cooked lobster chunks
12. Once the lobster is warmed through, remove from heat allow the dish to cool completely
13. Distribute among the containers, store for 2 days
14. To Serve: Reheat in the microwave for 1-2 min or until heated through. Garnish with parsley and enjoy!

Nutrition: Calories 752.5, Fat 12.5 g, Protein 67 g, Carbs 86 g, Fiber 2 g, Sugar 5 g

POTATO AND TUNA SALAD

18 minutes	0 minutes	4

INGREDIENTS

- 450 g baby potatoes, scrubbed, boiled
- 128 g tuna chunks, drained
- 128 g cherry tomatoes, halved
- 128 g medium onion, thinly sliced
- 8 pitted black olives
- 2 medium hard-boiled eggs, sliced
- 1 head Romaine lettuce
- Honey lemon mustard dressing
- 32 ml olive oil
- 2 tablespoons lemon juice
- 1 tablespoon Dijon mustard
- 1 teaspoon dill weed, chopped
- Salt as needed
- Pepper as needed

DIRECTIONS

1. Take a small glass bowl and mix in your olive oil, honey, lemon juice, Dijon mustard and dill
2. Season the mix with pepper and salt
3. Add in the tuna, baby potatoes, cherry tomatoes, red onion, green beans, black olives and toss everything nicely
4. Arrange your lettuce leaves on a beautiful serving dish to make the base of your salad
5. Top them up with your salad mixture and place the egg slices
6. Drizzle it with the previously prepared Salad Dressing
7. Serve

Nutrition: Calories 287.5, Fat 16.5 g, Protein 28 g, Carbs 21 g, Fiber 2.5 g, Sugar 2.5 g

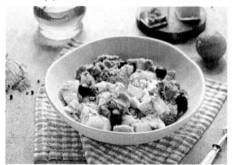

SKILLET BRAISED COD WITH ASPARAGUS AND POTATOES

20 minutes

20 minutes

4

INGREDIENTS

- 4 skinless cod fillets
- 450 g asparagus
- 340 g halved small purple potatoes
- Finely grated zest of ½ lemon
- Juice of ½ lemon
- 64 ml white wine
- 32 g torn fresh basil leaves
- 1 ½ tbsp. olive oil
- 1 tbsp. capers
- 3 cloves sliced garlic

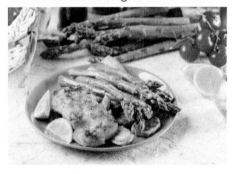

DIRECTIONS

1. Take a large and tall pan on the sides and heat the oil over medium-high.
2. Season the cod abundantly with salt and pepper and put in the pan, with the hot oil, for 1 min.
3. Carefully flip for 1 more min and after transferring the cod to a plate set it aside.
4. Add the lemon zest, capers and garlic to the pan and mix to coat with the remaining oil in the pan and cook about 1 minute. Fill in the wine and deglaze the pan.
5. Add lemon juice, potatoes, ½ tsp salt, ¼ tsp pepper and 250 ml of water and boil, decrease heat and simmer for 11 min.
6. Mix the asparagus and cook for 2 min.
7. Bring back the cod filets and any juices accumulated in the pan and cook until the asparagus are tender, for about 3 min.
8. Divide the cod fillets into shallow bowls and add the potatoes and asparagus and mix the basil in the broth left in the pan and pour over the cod.

Nutrition: Calories 314.5, Fat 6.5 g, Protein 44 g, Carbs 17 g, Fiber 4 g, Sugar 2.5 g

TUNA WITH VEGETABLE MIX

8 minutes

16 minutes

4

INGREDIENTS

- 32 ml extra-virgin olive oil, divided
- 1 tablespoon rice vinegar
- 1 teaspoon kosher salt, divided
- ¾ teaspoon Dijon mustard
- ¾ teaspoon honey
- 115 g baby gold beets, thinly sliced
- 115 g fennel bulb, trimmed and thinly sliced
- 115 g baby turnips, thinly sliced
- 170 g Granny Smith apple, very thinly sliced
- 2 teaspoons sesame seeds, toasted
- 170 g tuna steaks
- ½ teaspoon black pepper
- 1 tablespoon fennel fronds, torn

DIRECTIONS

1. Scourge 2 tablespoons of oil, ½ a teaspoon of salt, honey, vinegar, and mustard.
2. Give the mixture a nice mix.
3. Add fennel, beets, apple, and turnips; mix and toss until everything is evenly coated.
4. Sprinkle with sesame seeds and toss well.
5. Using cast-iron skillet, heat 2 tablespoons of oil over high heat.
6. Carefully season the tuna with ½ a teaspoon of salt and pepper
7. Situate the tuna in the skillet and cook for 4 min, giving 1½ min per side.
8. Remove the tuna and slice it up.
9. Place in containers with the vegetable mix.
10. Serve with the fennel mix, and enjoy!

Nutrition: Calories 209, Fat 15 g, Protein 12 g, Carbs 4 g, Fiber 1 g, Sugar 2 g

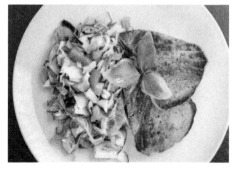

PEPPER SALMON SKEWERS

25 minutes

15 minutes

5

INGREDIENTS

- 680 g salmon fillet
- 64 g Plain yogurt
- 1 teaspoon paprika
- 1 teaspoon turmeric
- 1 teaspoon red pepper
- 1 teaspoon salt
- 1 teaspoon dried cilantro
- 1 teaspoon sunflower oil
- ½ teaspoon ground nutmeg

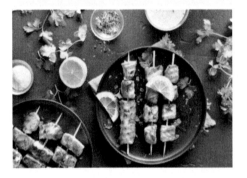

DIRECTIONS

1. For the marinade: mix up together Plain yogurt, paprika, turmeric red pepper, salt, and ground nutmeg.
2. Chop the salmon fillet roughly and put it in the yogurt mixture.
3. Mix up well and marinate for 25 minutes.
4. Then skew the fish on the skewers.
5. Sprinkle the skewers with sunflower oil and place in the tray.
6. Bake the salmon skewers for 15 minutes at 190 C.

Nutrition: Calories 211.5, Fat 9 g, Protein 35.5 g, Carbs 2 g, Fiber 0 g, Sugar 1.5 g

TOMATO GREEK SALAD

15 minutes

0 minutes

4

INGREDIENTS

- 450 g tomatoes, cubed
- 1 cucumber, sliced
- 64 g black olives
- 32 g sun-dried tomatoes, chopped
- 1 red onion, sliced
- 32 g parsley, chopped
- Salt and pepper to taste
- 1 tablespoon balsamic vinegar
- 2 tablespoons extra virgin olive oil

DIRECTIONS

1. Combine the tomatoes, cucumber, black olives, sun-dried tomatoes, onion and parsley in a bowl.
2. Add salt and pepper to taste then stir in the vinegar and olive oil.
3. Mix well and serve the salad fresh.

Nutrition: Calories: 126, Fat: 9.2 g, Protein: 2.1 g, Carbohydrates: 11.5 g

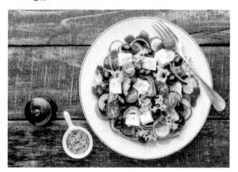

GREEN MEDITERRANEAN SALAD

15 minutes

0 minutes

4

INGREDIENTS

- 256 g arugula leaves
- 256 g baby spinach
- 2 cucumbers, sliced
- 2 celery stalks, sliced
- 64 g chopped parsley
- 32 g chopped cilantro
- 1 lemon, juiced
- 1 tablespoon balsamic vinegar
- Salt and pepper to taste

DIRECTIONS

1. Combine the arugula and spinach with the rest of the ingredients in a salad bowl.
2. Add salt and pepper to taste and season well with salt and pepper.
3. Serve the salad fresh.

Nutrition: Calories 32, Fat 0 g, Protein 1 g, Carbs 6.5 g, Fiber 2.5 g, Sugar 5 g

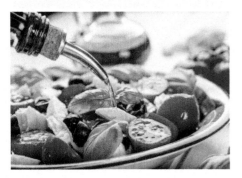

MEDITERRANEAN VEGGIE BOWL

10 minutes

20 minutes

4

INGREDIENTS

- 128 g quinoa, rinsed
- 1½ teaspoons salt, divided
- 256 g cherry tomatoes, cut in half
- 1 large bell pepper, cucumber
- 128 g Kalamata olives

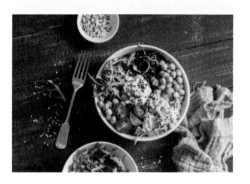

DIRECTIONS

1. Using medium pot over medium heat, boil 250 ml of water. Add the bulgur (or quinoa) and 1 teaspoon of salt. Close and cook for 18 min.
2. To arrange the veggies in your 4 bowls, visually divide each bowl into 5 sections. Place the cooked bulgur in one section. Follow with the tomatoes, bell pepper, cucumbers, and olives.
3. Scourge 64 ml of lemon juice, olive oil, remaining ½ teaspoon salt, and black pepper.
4. Evenly spoon the dressing over the 4 bowls.
5. Serve.

Nutrition: Calories 205.5, Fat 5 g, Protein 7 g, Carbs 33 g, Fiber 4 g, Sugar 3.5 g

CHICKPEA PITA PATTIES

12 minutes

21 minutes

4

INGREDIENTS

- 1 egg, large
- 2 teaspoons oregano
- 64 g panko bread crumbs, whole wheat
- sea salt & black pepper to taste
- 1 tablespoon olive oil
- 1 cucumber, halved lengthwise
- 170 g Greek yogurt, 2%
- clove garlic, minced
- 4 pita bread, whole wheat & halved
- 1 tomato, cut into 4 thick slices
- 64 g hummus
- 425 g chickpeas, drained & rinsed

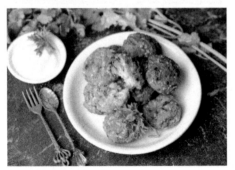

DIRECTIONS

1. Get out a large bowl, mash your chickpeas with a potato masher, and then add in your bread crumbs, eggs, hummus, oregano, and pepper. Stir well. Form four patties, and then press them flat on a plate. They should be 2 cm thick.
2. Get out a skillet, placing it over medium-high heat. Heat the oil until hot, which should take three min. Cook the patties for five min per side.
3. While your patties are cooking, shred half of your cucumber with a grader, and then stir your shredded cucumber, garlic, and yogurt together to make a tzatziki sauce. Slice the remaining cucumber into slices that are a 0.5 cm thick before placing them to the side.
4. Toast your pita bread, and then assemble your sandwich with each one having a tomato slice, a few slices of cucumber, chickpea patty, and drizzle each one with your sauce to serve.

Nutrition: Calories 621, Fat 13.5 g, Protein 27.5 g, Carbs 96 g, Fiber 14 g, Sugar 12 g

CHICKPEA SALAD MOROCCAN STYLE

15 minutes

0 minutes

6

INGREDIENTS

- 42.5 g crumbled low-fat feta cheese
- 32 g fresh mint, chopped
- 32 g fresh cilantro, chopped
- 1 red bell pepper, diced
- 2 plum tomatoes, diced
- 3 green onions, sliced thinly
- 1 large carrot, peeled and julienned
- 384 g BPA free canned chickpeas or garbanzo beans
- Pinch of cayenne pepper
- ¼ tsp salt
- ¼ tsp pepper
- 2 tsp ground cumin
- 3 tbsp fresh lemon juice
- 3 tbsp olive oil

DIRECTIONS

1. Make the dressing by whisking cayenne, black pepper, salt, cumin, lemon juice and oil in a small bowl and set aside.
2. Mix together feta, mint, cilantro, red pepper, tomatoes, onions, carrots and chickpeas in a large salad bowl.
3. Pour now dressing over salad and toss to coat well.
4. Serve and enjoy.

Nutrition: Calories 300; Protein: 13.2g; Carbs: 35.4g; Fat: 12.8g

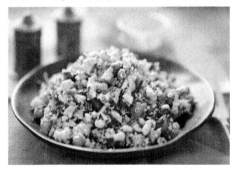

SUN-DRIED TOMATOES AND CHICKPEAS

15 minutes

10 minutes

6

INGREDIENTS

- 1 red bell pepper
- 64 g parsley, chopped
- 32 ml red wine vinegar
- 2 410 g cans chickpeas, drained and rinsed
- 2 cloves garlic, chopped
- 256 ml water
- 2 tablespoons extra-virgin olive oil
- 4 sun-dried tomatoes
- Salt to taste

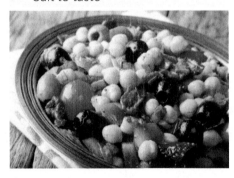

DIRECTIONS

1. Lengthwise, slice bell pepper in half. Place on baking sheet with skin side up. Broil on top rack for 5 minutes until skin is blistered.
2. In a brown paper bag, place the charred bell pepper halves. Fold bag and leave in there for 10 minutes. Remove pepper and peel off skin. Slice into thin strips.
3. Meanwhile, microwave 250 ml of water to boiling. Add the sun-dried tomatoes and leave in to reconstitute for 10 minutes. Drain and slice into thin strips.
4. Whisk well olive oil, garlic, and red wine vinegar.
5. Mix in parsley, sun-dried tomato, bell pepper, and chickpeas.
6. Season with salt to taste and serve.

Nutrition: Calories 195; Protein: 8.0g; Carbs: 26.0g; Fat: 7.0g

ZUCCHINI AND BROWN RICE

5 minutes

50 minutes

4 Cups

INGREDIENTS

- 2 TB. extra-virgin olive oil
- 2 large zucchini, diced
- 1 (455 g) can artichoke hearts, rinsed and drained
- 1 TB. fresh dill
- 1 tsp. ground black pepper
- 1 tsp. salt
- 512 ml chicken or vegetable broth
- 256 g basmati brown rice

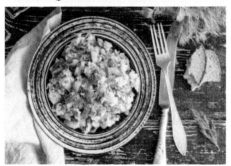

DIRECTIONS

1. In a large, 3-quart pot over medium heat, heat the extra-virgin olive oil. Add zucchini, and cook for 3 minutes.
2. Now add artichoke hearts, and cook for 2 minutes.
3. Add dill, black pepper, salt, and chicken broth, and bring to a simmer. Stir in basmati brown rice, cover, reduce heat to low, and cook for 40 minutes.
4. Remove from heat, uncover, fluff with a fork, cover, and let sit for another 15 minutes. Serve with Greek yogurt.

Nutrition: Calories 636, Fat 11 g, Protein 10 g, Carbs 117 g, Fiber 9 g, Sugar 5.5 g

BLACK BEANS AND QUINOA

10 minutes

30 minutes

6

INGREDIENTS

- 64 g chopped cilantro
- 2 cans black beans (425 g each), rinsed, drained
- 128 g frozen corn kernels
- Pepper and salt to taste
- ¼ tsp cayenne pepper
- 1 tsp ground cumin
- 192 ml vegetable broth
- 96 g quinoa
- 3 cloves garlic, chopped
- 1 onion, chopped
- 1 tsp vegetable oil

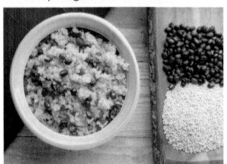

DIRECTIONS

1. On medium fire, place a saucepan and heat oil.
2. Add garlic and onions. Sauté for 5 minutes or until onions are soft.
3. Add quinoa. Pour vegetable broth and bring to a boil while increasing fire.
4. As you wait for broth to boil, season quinoa mixture with pepper, salt, cayenne pepper, and cumin.
5. Once boiling, reduce fire to a simmer, cover and simmer around 20 minutes or until liquid is fully absorbed.
6. Once liquid is fully absorbed, stir in black beans and frozen corn. Continue cooking until heated through, around 5 minutes.
7. To serve, add cilantro, toss well to mix, and enjoy.

Nutrition: Calories: 262; Carbs: 47.1g; Protein: 13.0g; Fat: 2.9g

ITALIAN WHITE BEAN SOUP

15 minutes

25 minutes

4

INGREDIENTS

- 1 (400 g) can chicken broth
- 1 bunch of fresh spinach, rinsed and thinly sliced
- 1 clove garlic, minced
- 1 stalk celery, chopped
- 1 tablespoon lemon juice
- 1 tablespoon vegetable oil
- 1 onion, chopped
- 1/4 teaspoon ground black pepper
- 1/8 teaspoon dried thyme
- 2 (455 g) cans of white kidney beans, rinsed, drained
- 256 ml water

DIRECTIONS

1. Place a pot on medium high fire and heat it for a minute. Add oil and heat for another minute.
2. Stir in celery and onion. Sauté for 7 minutes.
3. Stir in garlic and cook for another minute.
4. Add water, thyme, pepper, chicken broth, and beans. Cover and simmer for 15 minutes.
5. Remove half of the bean and celery mixture with a slotted spoon and set aside.
6. With an immersion blender, puree remaining soup in pot until smooth and creamy.
7. Return in the bean mixture previously set aside. Stir in spinach and lemon juice. Cook for 2 minutes until heated through and spinach is wilted.
8. Serve and enjoy.

Nutrition: Calories: 245; Protein: 12.0 g; Carbs: 38.1 g; Fat: 4.9 g

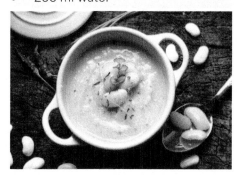

FLOURLESS CHOCOLATE CAKE

20 minutes

25 minutes

8

INGREDIENTS

- 226 g dark chocolate, chopped
- 113 g butter, cubed
- 6 eggs, separated
- 1 teaspoon vanilla extract
- 1 pinch salt
- 4 tablespoons white sugar
- Berries for serving

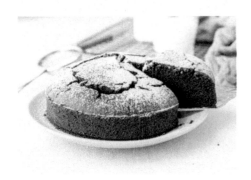

DIRECTIONS

1. Combine the chocolate and butter in a heatproof bowl and melt them together until smooth.
2. When smooth, remove off heat and place aside.
3. Separate the eggs.
4. Mix the egg yolks with the chocolate mixture.
5. Whip the egg whites with a pinch of salt until puffed up. Add the sugar and mix for a few more minutes until glossy and stiff.
6. Fold the meringue into the chocolate mixture then pour the batter in a 23 cm round cake pan lined with baking paper.
7. Bake in the preheated oven at 175 C for 25 minutes.
8. Serve the cake chilled.

Nutrition: Calories:324, Fat: 23.2 g, Protein: 6.4 g, Carbs: 23.2 g

YOGURT PANNA COTTA WITH FRESH BERRIES

15 minutes

4-5 Hours (Rest Time)

6

INGREDIENTS

- 256 g Greek yogurt
- 128 g milk
- 128 g heavy cream
- 2 teaspoons gelatin powder
- 4 tablespoons cold water
- 4 tablespoons honey
- 1 teaspoon vanilla extract
- 1 teaspoon lemon zest
- 1 pinch salt
- 256 g mixed berries for serving

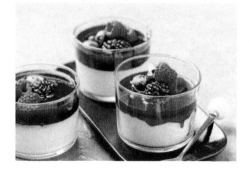

DIRECTIONS

1. Combine the milk and cream in a saucepan and heat them up.
2. Bloom the gelatin in cold water for 10 minutes.
3. Remove the milk off heat and stir in the gelatin until dissolved.
4. Add the vanilla, lemon zest and salt and allow to cool down.
5. Stir in the yogurt then pour the mixture into serving glasses.
6. Put in the fridge and when set, top with fresh berries and serve.

Nutrition: Calories 155.5, Fat 6 g, Protein 5.5 g, Carbs 19.5 g, Fiber 2 g, Sugar 17 g

MELON CUCUMBER SMOOTHIE

10 minutes

0 minutes

2

INGREDIENTS

- ½ cucumber
- 2 slices of melon
- 2 tablespoons lemon juice
- 1 pear, peeled and sliced
- 3 fresh mint leaves
- 64 ml almond milk

DIRECTIONS

1. Place all Ingredients in a blender.
2. Blend until smooth.
3. Pour in a glass container and allow to chill in the fridge for at least 30 minutes.

Nutrition: Calories 60, Fat 0.5 g, Protein 0 g, Carbs 13 g, Fiber 2 g, Sugar 7.5 g

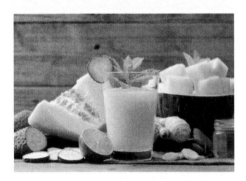

CINNAMON STUFFED PEACHES

10 minutes

5 minutes

4

INGREDIENTS

- 4 peaches, pitted, halved
- 2 tablespoons ricotta cheese
- 2 tablespoons of liquid honey
- 96 ml of water
- ½ teaspoon vanilla extract
- ¾ teaspoon ground cinnamon
- 1 tablespoon almonds, sliced
- ¾ teaspoon saffron

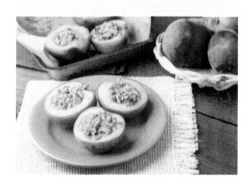

DIRECTIONS

1. Pour water in the saucepan and bring to boil.
2. Add vanilla extract, saffron, ground cinnamon, and liquid honey.
3. Cook the liquid until the honey is melted.
4. Then remove it from the heat.
5. Put the halved peaches in the hot honey liquid.
6. Meanwhile, make the filling: mix up together ricotta cheese, vanilla extract, and sliced almonds.
7. Remove the peaches from honey liquid and arrange in the plate.
8. Fill 4 peach halves with ricotta filling and cover them with remaining peach halves.
9. Sprinkle the cooked dessert with liquid honey mixture gently.

Nutrition: Calories 117.5, Fat 3 g, Protein 2 g, Carbs 21 g, Fiber 2 g, Sugar 19.5 g

MINTY TART

10 minutes

30 minutes

6

INGREDIENTS

- 128 g tart cherries, pitted
- 128 g wheat flour, whole grain
- 42.5 g butter, softened
- ½ teaspoon baking powder
- 1 tablespoon Erythritol
- ¼ teaspoon dried mint
- ¾ teaspoon salt

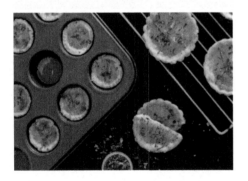

DIRECTIONS

1. Mix up together wheat flour and butter.
2. Add baking powder and salt. Knead the soft dough.
3. Then place the dough in the freezer for 10 minutes.
4. When the dough is solid, remove it from the freezer and grate with the help of the grater. Place ¼ part of the grated dough in the freezer.
5. Sprinkle the springform pan with remaining dough and place tart cherries on it.
6. Sprinkle the berries with Erythritol and dried mint and cover with ¼ part of dough from the freezer.
7. Bake the cake for 30 minutes at 185 C. The cooked tart will have a golden brown surface.

Nutrition: Calories 118, Fat 4.5 g, Protein 2.5 g, Carbs 19 g, Fiber 2.5 g, Sugar 3 g

DELECTABLE MANGO SMOOTHIE

5 minutes

0 minutes

2

INGREDIENTS

- 256 g diced mango
- 1 carrot, peeled and sliced roughly
- 1 orange, peeled and segmented
- Fresh mint leaves

DIRECTIONS

1. Place the mango, carrot, and oranges in a blender.
2. Pulse until smooth.
3. Pour now in a glass container and allow to chill before serving.
4. Garnish with mint leaves on top.

Nutrition: Calories 134; Carbs: 33.6g; Protein: 2g; Fat: 0.7g; Sugar

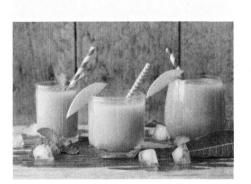

YOGURT SUNDAE

5 minutes

0 minutes

1

INGREDIENTS

- 96 g plain Greek yogurt
- 32 g fresh mixed berries (blueberries, strawberries, blackberries)
- 2 tablespoons walnut pieces
- 1 tablespoon ground flaxseed
- 2 fresh mint leaves, shredded

DIRECTIONS

1. Pour the yogurt into a tall parfait glass and sprinkle with the mixed berries, walnut pieces, and flaxseed.
2. Garnish with the shredded mint leaves and serve immediately.

Nutrition: Calories 278, Fat 15 g, Protein 14 g, Carbs 20 g, Fiber 3 g, Sugar 8 g

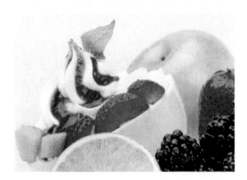

MEAL PLAN

DAY 1
Breakfast: Mediterranean Omelet p.12

Lunch: Tuna Pasta p.27

Dinner: Coconut Chicken p.39

Dessert: Yogurt Sundae p.70

DAY 2
Breakfast: Salmon Frittata p.13

Lunch: Vegetable risotto p.29

Dinner: Rosemary Pork Chops p.32

Dessert: Cinnamon Stuffed Peaches p.67

DAY 3
Breakfast: Creamy Oatmeal p.22

Lunch: Broccoli Pesto Spaghetti p.24

Dinner: Pepper Salmon Skewers p.54

Dessert: Yogurt Panna Cotta with Fresh Berries p.65

DAY 4
Breakfast: Paleo Almond Banana Pancakes p.22

Lunch: Beef Pitas p.35

Dinner: Seafood Paella p.50
Dessert: Minty Tart p.68

DAY 5
Breakfast: Stuffed Avocado p.17

Lunch: Mediterranean-Style Salmon Burgers p.26

Dinner: Stuffed Pork chops p.33

Dessert: Cinnamon Stuffed Peaches p.67

DAY 6
Breakfast: Salmon Frittata p.13

Lunch: Sun-dried Tomato Pesto Penne p.23

Dinner: Parsnip Chickpea Veal Stew p.28

Dessert: Flourless Chocolate Cake p.64

DAY 7
Breakfast: Zucchini Cakes p.15

Lunch: Coriander Shrimps p.49

Dinner: Creamy Salmon Soup p.30

Dessert: Melon Cucumber Smoothie p.66

DAY 8
Breakfast: Spiced Breakfast Casserole p.21

Lunch: Mediterranean-style Tuna Wrap p.25

Dinner: Vegetable risotto p.29

Dessert: Delectable Mango Smoothie p.69

DAY 9

Breakfast: Creamy Oatmeal p.22

Lunch: Fried Salmon p.48

Dinner: Chicken Quesadilla p.38

Dessert: Cinnamon Stuffed Peaches p.67

DAY 10

Breakfast: Mediterranean Omelet p.12

Lunch: Broccoli Pesto Spaghetti p.24

Dinner: Lamb and Rice p.31

Dessert: Yogurt Panna Cotta with Fresh Berries p.65

DAY 11

Breakfast: Tuna Salad p.11

Lunch: Basil Chicken with Olives p.43

Dinner: Seafood Paella p.50

Dessert: Flourless Chocolate Cake p.64

DAY 12

Breakfast: Italian Scrambled Eggs p.20

Lunch: Pork and Tomato Meatloaf p.37

Dinner: Tuna Pasta p.27

Dessert: Yogurt Sundae p.70

DAY 13

Breakfast: Creamy Oatmeal p.22

Lunch: Salmon and Mango Mix p.47

Dinner: Broccoli Pesto Spaghetti p.24

Dessert: Delectable Mango Smoothie p.69

DAY 14

Breakfast: Spiced Breakfast Casserole p.21

Lunch: Vegetable risotto p.29

Dinner: Chipotle Turkey And Tomatoes p.41

Dessert: Minty Tart p.68

CONVERSION TABLE

Volume Equivalents (Liquid)

US STANDARD
US STANDARD (OUNCES)
METRIC (APPROXIMATE)

2 tbsp
1 fl. oz.
30 mL

1/4 cup
2 fl. oz.
60 mL

1/2 cup
4 fl. oz.
120 mL

1 cup
8 fl. oz.
240 mL

11/2 cups
12 fl. oz.
355 mL

2 cups or 1 pint
16 fl. oz.
475 mL

4 cups or 1 quart
32 fl. oz.
1 L

1 gallon
128 fl. oz.

4 L

Volume Equivalents (Dry)

US STANDARD
METRIC (APPROXIMATE)

1/8 tsp
0.5 mL

1/4 tsp
1 mL

1/2 tsp
2 mL

3/4 tsp
4 mL

1 tsp
5 mL

1 tbsp
15 mL

1/4 cup
59 mL

1/3 cup
79 mL

1/2 cup
118 mL

2/3 cup

156 mL	120°C
3/4 cup	**300°F**
177 mL	150°C
1 cup	**325°F**
235 mL	165°C
2 cups or 1 pint	**350°F**
475 mL	180°C
3 cups	**375°F**
700 mL	190°C
4 cups or 1 quart	**400°F**
1 L	200°C

Oven Temperatures

FAHRENHEIT (F)
CELSIUS (C) (APPROXIMATE)

425°F	
220°C	
450°F	
250°F	230°C

INDEX

Printed in Great Britain
by Amazon

10454044R00045